THE IMPACT OF SEX IN A RELATIONHIP

By

Robert H. Rio

Table of Contents

Introduction

Sex has long been regarded as a necessary component of a love relationship. It's capable of strengthening emotional ties and fostering intimacy between lovers. If handled improperly, sex can also have a negative effect on a relationship. Misunderstandings, a breakdown in communication, and irritation may result. Conflicts may arise when the expectations and desires of the couple disagree. Additionally, sex-related issues like erectile dysfunction or a partner's lack of sexual interest can be upsetting and frustrating. The connection can be improved and strengthened via effective communication and mutual understanding of one another's needs and wants. If both partners are willing to discuss and compromise, sex can improve a relationship.

We will look at the effects sex has on relationships in this book.

Sex is a crucial component of physical closeness in a relationship, according to Chapter 1 of the book. It can strengthen their physical connection and aid in the emotional bonding of couples.

A good sex life depends on effective communication, which is discussed in Chapter 2. It might enhance your sexual experience and enrich your connection to discuss your preferences, needs, and wishes with your spouse.

Chapter 3: Mutual respect and trust are essential components of a good sexual relationship. Couples who trust one another are more inclined to open up about their sexual thoughts and desires, which results in a more satisfying sex life.

Sex may be a fantastic stress reliever, easing tension and anxiety in a relationship (Chapter 4). Additionally, it promotes the release of feel-good hormones like oxytocin, which can elevate mood and aid in relaxation.

Chapter 5: Health Benefits Regular sexual activity can enhance heart health, reduce stress, and boost immune system function, among other health advantages. A good sex life can also improve general well-being and self-esteem.

Chapter 1: Physical Closeness

It is both a basic human want and a requirement for establishing a stable connection. It is essential for forging a solid emotional connection and fostering an atmosphere of trust and closeness between partners. Sex is a potent manifestation of physical closeness in a love relationship that can have a big impact on how the partnership functions as a whole.

A greater level of connection between lovers can be formed through sex. The "love hormone" oxytocin is one of the hormones that are released during sexual intercourse between two people. This hormone promotes emotional connection, trust-building, and stress reduction. Because of this, having sex can assist to deepen the emotional bond between partners and raise their degree of contentment and enjoyment in the union as a whole.

However, it is impossible to ignore how having sex can harm a relationship. Physical closeness is an ongoing process that needs to be regularly cultivated; it is not a one-time occurrence. One partner may feel emotionally distant, less confident, and less affectionate toward the other when they are not happy with the level of physical closeness.

Additionally, having too much or too little sex can cause irritation and disappointment. Partners may start to take each other for granted if there is too much sex between them because they will have grown accustomed to one another. On the other hand, a lack of sex or physical closeness might cause rejection feelings and a decline in overall relationship satisfaction. When this occurs, a couple should make sure to talk about the importance of physical intimacy and establish open lines of communication.

In conclusion, sex and physical intimacy have a significant impact on the nature and viability of any love partnership. To keep a healthy relationship, it's critical to foster both the partners' physical and emotional ties. To maintain a healthy and satisfying level of physical intimacy, communication and respect between partners are essential. Therefore, in order to maintain a strong and happy relationship, partners should be aware of

their emotional and physical needs, stay
in touch, and put forth constant effort.

Chapter 2: Communication

It is impossible to stress the importance of communication in a loving relationship. It is essential for creating closeness, trust, and a stronger emotional connection between partners. The need for communication increases when considering how sex affects a relationship. Although talking about sex might be difficult, it's important to be open and honest about it.

Relationship sex can affect communication in a number of different ways. Regular sexual activity between couples may find that the intimacy and connection that comes with it helps create greater communication. Deep chats, honest discussions, and the building blocks of a successful relationship are frequently sparked by being vulnerable and intimate with one another. Additionally, sharing one another's emotional and physical needs makes it easier for couples to communicate their true feelings to one another.

Lack of communication regarding sex, however, can result in misunderstandings and disappointments, endangering the stability of a partnership. One of the partners may feel unsatisfied, unwanted, or even rejected if they prefer more sex than the other. It's imperative to have an open discussion about each other's bodily requirements, desires, and boundaries in order to determine whether they are on the same page. It is crucial to discuss this issue together and look into alternative types of closeness that can be more rewarding and fulfilling if one partner is uncomfortable or unwilling to engage in sex.

In relationships that call for open and honest communication, sexual issues like performance anxiety or trouble eliciting an orgasm also frequently surface. Such situations require a great deal of patience, compassion, and empathy. A safe, judgment-free environment should be established between partners so that they may discuss their issues openly and work together to find solutions.

Let's sum up by saying that communication is a crucial component of any relationship and that sex can have a significant impact on it. Establishing a place where partners can discuss their emotional and physical desires, set boundaries, and work to create a meaningful, comfortable setting is crucial.

Therefore, openness, honesty, and trust are developed in a relationship through regular discussion of sex, which results in a healthier and happier union.

Chapter 3: Belief

Any connection that succeeds is built on trust. It serves as a foundation for emotional connection, vulnerability, and intimacy. For many couples, having sex is essential to establishing and preserving trust. Trust can be strengthened by a satisfying sexual connection, whereas it can be destroyed by sexual problems or betrayals. I'll talk about how sex affects a relationship's level of trust in this essay.

Between lovers, sex can foster an emotional sense of intimacy and connection. Sexual activity between couples helps them develop emotional trust, and this trust is frequently increased outside of the bedroom. Sharing one's body with someone involves a lot of vulnerability and trust. It strengthens their commitment to one another and cultivates a stronger sense of trust when both partners are open and honest about their physical and emotional desires.

But sexual betrayal can also negatively affect trust. Relationships can suffer a great deal from betrayals like adultery, and it can take time and effort to regain trust. A partner's trust can be destroyed by infidelity, leaving them feeling vulnerable and uneasy in the relationship. Before engaging in sexual activity, it is crucial to have an honest discussion about sexual boundaries in order to avoid any such betrayals.

Furthermore, trust levels can also be impacted by a partner's sexual history. The current partnership may suffer from insecurities and mistrust if one person has had previous sexual relationships. Both partners should be open and honest about their sexual preferences and concerns. A couple can overcome their concerns and increase their level of trust by talking about these things.

Healthy sexual interaction can also increase trust in a partnership. One partner may feel uneasy and insecure about broaching the subject if they are not satisfied with the sexual aspects of their relationship. Sexual desires can be spoken in an atmosphere where both lovers feel safe, heard, and acknowledged, thus fostering a sense of trust between them.

In conclusion, trust in a relationship is significantly impacted by sex. Through emotional closeness, a satisfying sexual relationship can increase trust, but sexual betrayals can erode it. To establish a secure, open environment that fosters trust, it is imperative to discuss openly and honestly about sexual preferences. Couples may create and retain trust and promote a healthy, rewarding sexual connection by being honest, empathic, and patient.

Chapter 4: Managing Stress

The pace of modern life frequently leads to high levels of stress, and it can be challenging to successfully manage it. Stress is a typical problem that many people experience. Sex in this situation, especially in the context of a healthy romantic relationship, can significantly improve stress alleviation.

The endorphins released during sex are one of the main ways it might reduce stress. Endorphins are organic substances that the body produces while engaged in specific activities including exercise, laughter, and sexual activity.

Cortisol and other stress hormones are known to be reduced by endorphins, which can increase feelings of relaxation and well-being. Therefore, if both couples consciously choose to emphasize it as part of their daily routine, sexual engagement can be a potent strategy to manage stress in a relationship.

Additionally, having sex can improve sleep quality and lower anxiety, both of which are important for controlling stress levels. Stress can be significantly exacerbated by anxiety, which can also start a vicious cycle of unfavorable thoughts and emotions. People can have a little break from these emotions and feel more at ease by having sexual activity. This may then spill over into other aspects of their lives, resulting in improved sleep, more productivity, and improved interactions with others.

It should be mentioned that sex has considerable stress-relieving effects when it takes place in a loving and supportive relationship. According to a Carnegie Mellon University study, those who have a spouse who is supportive during stressful times are less likely to get sick than people who are single. A relationship's foundation may be strengthened through sex, which will increase emotional support and stability.

In conclusion, one of the numerous advantages that sex may provide to a partnership is stress reduction. Sex can have a big impact on a couple's capacity to handle stress and sustain a successful relationship by generating endorphins, lowering anxiety, and fostering better sleep. However, it's crucial to keep in mind that sex is not a solution to every issue in life. To really enjoy this personal activity, it is essential to address underlying issues and make sure that a relationship is marked by honest communication, empathy, and respect. Numerous physical and mental health advantages of sexual engagement have been demonstrated, and these advantages might be especially obvious in the setting of a healthy relationship. The primary health advantages of engaging in sexual activity within a committed relationship will be discussed in this article.

The ability of sexual engagement to maintain healthy levels of hormones like estrogen and testosterone is one of its key physical benefits. These hormones play a crucial role in many body processes, such as bone density, muscle mass, and cognitive ability. Regular sexual activity can also enhance blood circulation and flow, which reduces the risk of heart disease, stroke, and other circulatory diseases.

Chapter 5: Benefits to Health

A good sexual life has been associated with improved mental health outcomes, such as lower levels of anxiety and depression. This is probably because of the endorphin release that takes place during sexual activity, which can result in emotions of joy, relaxation, and well-being. Regular sexual engagement can also boost self-confidence and self-esteem, which can result in a more positive self-image and higher levels of overall life satisfaction.

The ability of sexual activity within a partnership to foster emotional closeness and intimacy is a significant health advantage. A sensation of connection and intimacy that results from the production of oxytocin during sexual activity might improve a relationship's sense of security and support. This can be especially helpful while going through stressful times or trying times in a relationship because it reduces loneliness and isolation sensations.

Another significant factor that contributes to general health and well-being is sexual engagement, which has the potential to be a potent stress-relieving technique. Sexual activity can help to relieve stress and encourage relaxation, which can help one feel refreshed and at ease. The emotional connection that results from sexual activity can also provide people with a sense of security and comfort, which can help them cope with daily challenges and have a more balanced, healthy life.

In conclusion, having sex in a committed relationship has a variety of positive effects on one's health. Sexual activity can help people feel happier, more fulfilled, and more connected within their relationships. It can also have positive effects on one's physical and mental health, including better hormone and circulatory function, as well as decreased levels of anxiety and sadness. As a result, maintaining a positive, active sexual relationship with a partner can be essential to one's overall health and well-being.

Conclusion

There is no denying the importance of sex in a loving relationship. Couples become more emotionally and physically connected when they show their love physically. The relationships between two people in a romantic relationship are clearly strengthened by sex, despite the fact that many people regard emotional fit, intimacy, trust, and respect as important relationship-building blocks.

When done properly, sex aids partners in discovering one other's needs, wants, and fantasies. Couples can develop intimacy, share vulnerable times, and have better communication thanks to it. In addition to aiding in stress reduction, a good sexual life also supports a strong immune system. In essence, sex is essential for both physical pleasure and general emotional and mental health.

A lack of sex or unsatisfied sexual cravings, however, can result in irritation and resentment, which can ultimately have a detrimental effect on the quality of the relationship. To ensure that both partners are pleased, it is essential for couples to openly communicate their sexual wants and aspirations. It is also crucial to remember that sex should always be voluntary and never employed as a means of control or compulsion.

In summary, sex is an important aspect of any relationship. In addition to fostering overall well-being, it can aid in the emotional and physical closeness of couples. To promote sexual fulfillment, however, it is crucial that partners talk frankly about their desires, respect one another's boundaries, and cooperate.